Carb Cycling Guide

Learn How to Lose Weight and Build Muscle While Still Enjoying Carbs

By Nathan Hollister

© **Copyright 2020 - All rights reserved.**

The content contained within this book may not be reproduced, duplicated or transmitted without direct written permission from the author or the publisher.

Under no circumstances will any blame or legal responsibility be held against the publisher or author for any damages, reparation, or monetary loss due to the information contained within this book. Either directly or indirectly.

Legal Notice:

This book is copyright protected. This book is only for personal use. You cannot amend, distribute, sell, use, quote or paraphrase any part, or the content within this book, without the consent of the author or publisher.

Disclaimer Notice:

Please note the information contained within this document is for educational and entertainment purposes only. All effort has been executed to present accurate, up to date and reliable, complete information. No warranties of any kind are declared or implied. Readers acknowledge that the author is not engaging in the rendering of legal, financial, medical or professional advice. The content within this book has been derived from various sources. Please consult a licensed professional before attempting any techniques outlined in this book.

By reading this document, the reader agrees that under no circumstances is the author responsible for any losses, direct or indirect, which are incurred as a result of the use of information contained within this document, including, but not limited to, —errors, omissions, or inaccuracies.

Contents

Introduction 1
   What Is Carbohydrate Cycling? 1
Chapter 1: Carbohydrate Cycling Benefits 3
   Am I a Bodybuilder? 8
   Should Everyone Do Carb Cycling? 10
Chapter 2: What Does Carbohydrate Cycling Involve? 14
   The Fundamentals 14
   Is Carbohydrate Cycling Like Keto? 16
Chapter 3: A Carbohydrate Cycling Diet Plan? 20
   High Carbohydrate Day 20
   Low Carbohydrate Day 22
   A Week-Long Carbohydrate Cycling Program 23
Chapter 4: Carbohydrate Cycling and Losing Weight 33
Chapter 5: Additional Advantages of Carbohydrate Cycling 37
Chapter 6: Things to Remember 39
   Customize It To Your Liking 40
   Protein and Calories 43
Chapter 7: Carbohydrate Cycling Types 46
Chapter 8: Which Foods Are Should You Be Eating? 51
   Carbs That Are Good For You 51
Chapter 9: Sample Programs 61
Chapter 10: How to Begin 73

Conclusion...81

Thank you for buying this book and I hope that you will find it useful. If you will want to share your thoughts on this book, you can do so by leaving a review on the Amazon page, it helps me out a lot.

Introduction

What Is Carbohydrate Cycling?

Carbohydrates, often called carbs, are a continuous hot subject now. Some dietary professionals are beginning to link them with issues like diabetes, inflammation and weight problems. Nevertheless, others continue to assert that they are a crucial part of our everyday eating plan. So, are all carbs bad for you? And how many carbs should you consume daily? This is where carb-cycling can assist.

Carbohydrates, in addition to protein and fat, comprise the 3 macronutrients. When your body absorbs carbs, they're broken down into glucose-- your brain and body's favored kind of fuel. When glucose enters into the blood stream, the pancreas is set off to generate a hormone referred to as insulin. This transfers glucose from the blood stream into the cell. Here, it is developed into energy, saved in the fat cells or stocked as glycogen.

When you start a carb-cycling program, you can decrease body fat while boosting muscle mass. It's an incredibly extensive eating plan, so it ought to just be utilized in the short-term. Nevertheless, it works for crushing weight-loss plateaus.

Carb cycling depends on reducing and increasing carbohydrate consumption on various days of the week. There are low-carb and high-carb days along with days on which no carbohydrates are eaten at all. When you attempt carbohydrate cycling, you can consume carbs in case they're from a clean source. The cycling enables the body to utilize fats as a fuel rather than burning carbohydrates and muscle.

In this book, we'll take a better look at what carbohydrate cycling is everything about. We'll check out how you can get going and how to identify whether it's right for you. This is going to permit you to make an educated decision.

Chapter 1: Carbohydrate Cycling Benefits

Carbohydrate cycling isn't perfect for everybody. Nevertheless, it can prove to be a helpful option in the appropriate conditions. There are 2 primary groups of individuals who can take advantage of trying this eating program: Those who have to slim down, and those who wish to increase their muscle mass while improving their sporting effectiveness.

Some specialists recommend that carbohydrate cycling is specifically useful for anybody who needs to slim down. In theory, this manner of eating can assist you to keep your physical functionality. It likewise offers a lot of the similar advantages offered by low-carb eating plans like the Atkins program. These types of eating plans can leave dieters feeling weak and sluggish. For that reason, carbohydrate cycling provides a clear benefit.

Like any other eating plan, the main system behind reducing weight is to preserve a deficit of calories. You have to consume less food than the body can burn over a prolonged duration. When you embrace carbohydrate cycling in addition to a deficit in calorie consumption, you'll probably drop weight.

Carbs aren't bad for you. Nevertheless, the duty of carbohydrates is to provide an energy source for your body to burn through when you're active. If you aren't performing enough physical activity and are still consuming a great deal of carbs, issues occur. Your body winds up keeping the excess as fat.

Carbohydrates are a terrific option when you're exercising hard in the gym. Your body is going to burn quickly through them to generate energy. It burns carbohydrates instead of protein, so this nutrient can improve muscle development. If you aren't training hard, those additional carbohydrates aren't being burned up rapidly. For that reason, the body keeps all the unused glucose in the fat cells. This leads to you ending up being overweight and even obese.

On the other hand, if you limit carbohydrate consumption, your body can not save the excess glucose. Rather, it resorts to fats to produce energy instead of sweet or starchy foods. Because of this, your body can shed fat, assisting you to slim down. Hoarding extra calories is all well and good if you have an extremely active way of life. Yet, if you aren't getting around much, you can not utilize all those calories. This results in weight problems. You, for that reason, have to vary your carbohydrate consumption from day to day. If you're going to be going to the gym, you can consume more carbohydrates. If you're going to be sitting in front of the television for the majority of the day, you ought to limit your consumption.

Another reason that carbohydrate cycling is so helpful for weight reduction is due to the fact that it makes it tough to overindulge. Foods with a high carbohydrate count are typically more indulgent. All of us understand how tough it is to withstand the urge to snack on another cookie or a tasty, sweet donut. It's a lot more difficult to binge eat on proteins and veggies. Extremely few individuals are going to over-indulge on broccoli or chicken! For that reason, you'll be consuming less calories and assisting your midsection.

As carbohydrate cycling is a versatile eating plan, it could be more interesting to dieters. Understanding that you can delight in carbohydrates sometimes could be appealing. Among the reasons that numerous individuals fall short with other eating plans is due to their limiting nature. Knowing you can never ever consume bread or pasta could be off-putting from the start. This results in dieters quitting after a short while. Carbohydrate cycling's versatility can motivate these individuals to stick to the program. Consequently, they'll lose more weight long-term and preserve a much healthier body weight.

There is additionally an essential link in between levels of insulin in the blood and carbohydrate consumption. If there is a high level of insulin in the blood, fat storage ends up being most likely. In turn, this impedes successful weight reduction. You ought to be cautious about altering your carbohydrate consumption if you're taking insulin for diabetes. For that reason, speaking to a medical professional is essential.

Healthy eating needs to additionally lie at the heart of any carbohydrate cycling program. It isn't a reason to limit eating to excess or over-indulge on junk food. Careful tracking is needed to be effective at carbohydrate cycling. This can promote an unhealthy mindset towards eating. For that reason, you have to make sure to stay in perspective when embracing this program. If you discover it's adversely impacting your life by doing this, you ought to stop and select a different eating program.

Am I a Bodybuilder?

Carbohydrate cycling is a popular nutrition approach for bodybuilders and athletes. Those who are physique competitors are specifically fond of this manner of eating. They depend greatly on no or low carbohydrate days in their contest preparation cutting stage. Because glycogen is mostly water, controling your carbohydrate consumption alters the look of muscles on stage. On the other hand, developing a surplus of energy by taking in more carbohydrates promotes much better muscle gain.

Numerous athletes utilize their method of eating to decrease their fat gain and optimize their muscle gain throughout training. They need to strictly abide by an everyday menu which is based upon their body structure and energy output. Additionally, a carbohydrate cycling program is going to control the quantity of proteins and fats being taken in.

A greater protein consumption is needed to promote muscle development throughout carbohydrate cycling. Protein needs to, for that reason, be approximately 30 percent of everyday calorie consumption. Carbohydrates in a low stage ought to be approximately 15 percent of overall consumption. These ought to mainly be made up of fresh veggies. High carbohydrate days ought to fall on days of extreme training. This is going to make sure muscle healing is quicker and vital nutrients are offered.

By having actually targeted carbohydrate intakes and routine durations of high carbohydrates, your functionality can enhance. For athletes taking part in endurance sports like cycling, swimming and running, this is excellent news. Varying carbohydrate consumption through the year assists to boost reserves of muscle glycogen.

Carbohydrate cycling enhances the carbohydrate load, so there's ample fuel to burn when exercising intensively. However, excess carbohydrates will not be kept as far when you're having a non-workout day. Elite athletes have actually been eating in this manner for a long time. They think it aids them to improve their exercise functionality. Simultaneously, they can build muscle while keeping a healthy body weight.

Athletes and bodybuilders who carb cycle additionally have much shorter recuperation times. Their glycogen replenishment gets an increase. Consequently, they can delight in much better gains in the gym.

Should Everyone Do Carb Cycling?

Sadly, carbohydrate cycling isn't the answer for everybody. In theory, it ought to be an appropriate method of eating for anybody. Nevertheless, some individuals fall short to carry it out appropriately. This might induce health issues and continuous problems.

When you follow any limiting diet plan, you have to be knowledgeable about when it's time to stop. If you continuously yearn for foods that are "off-limits" and feel bad if you indulge, this is a warning sign. Additionally, if you discover that carbohydrate cycling is adversely impacting your mindset and state of mind, this might be an issue. It's an indication that this isn't for you. Additionally, if you're abnormally tired when carbohydrate cycling, this is an indication to stop.

Anybody who has a history of eating conditions ought to stay clear of carbohydrate cycling. Limitation and adherence, along with tracking, measuring and counting are crucial elements of this eating plan. Continuously being aware of calorie and carbohydrate consumption strengthens disordered eating patterns. This can aggravate eating disorders and induce brand-new problems to establish.

Individuals who have particular medical conditions ought to stay clear of carbohydrate cycling. Individuals who have mood disorders like anxiety and depression might be negatively impacted. Altering eating patterns can cause even worse mood swings.

Individuals struggling with other medical conditions like cardiovascular disease and metabolic syndrome ought to additionally beware. This additionally applies to those struggling with diabetes. Although carbohydrate cycling could be great for controlling insulin levels, it could be bothersome for those on medication. If you're taking insulin for diabetes currently, you need to speak with your physician prior to attempting this diet plan. Falling short to do this might cause harmful outcomes for your total health and wellness.

Some other individuals ought to additionally stay clear of carbohydrate cycling. Ladies who are pregnant, for instance, ought to stay clear of any diet plan of this type. They have to have a consistent, continuous supply of carbs that are abundant in fiber to stay healthy. For the identical reason, breastfeeding moms ought to additionally stay away from this dietary program.

Nevertheless, when carbohydrate cycling is followed appropriately, it ought to be an appropriate method of eating for everybody. Numerous dieters discover the versatility of this routine fits their choices. They can still delight in carbohydrates sometimes and this makes them feel less limited. They additionally frequently discover that the tediousness of a routine eating plan is lowered.

It's for that reason typically suggested that you consult your medical professional prior to attempting carbohydrate cycling. A physician is going to have the ability to recommend whether it's an excellent option for you.

Chapter 2: What Does Carbohydrate Cycling Involve?

Understanding the science behind why carbohydrate cycling works is necessary for anybody thinking about embracing this routine. Without comprehending the principles of this eating plan, it's hard to follow it properly. Here, we take a look at the fundamentals.

The Fundamentals

Carbohydrate cycling is reasonably new in regards to dietary techniques. It is supported by science, based upon carb manipulation's biological systems. Yet, there are a couple of formal research studies which have actually specifically examined carbohydrate cycling eating plans. Lots of people have actually found this routine an effective one, nevertheless. Elite professional athletes have actually been utilizing this approach for many years to increase their effectiveness. Dieters are additionally beginning to acknowledge the advantages.

So, how does carbohydrate cycling work? Basically, this manner of eating intends to match up the body's needs for calories or glucose. For example, it provides carbs on days of extreme training or exercises. High carb days refuel glycogen in the muscles. This, too, can decrease the breakdown of the muscles and enhance sporting efficiency.

When high-carbohydrate durations are prepared strategically, it's possible to increase the performance of appetite-regulating hormones. Leptin and ghrelin are both hormones connected with appetite and hunger. Both could be much better managed with carbohydrate cycling eating plans.

On low carb days, the body changes to another method of generating energy. Without the glucose from carbohydrates to sustain it, it primarily starts to burn fat. This, consequently, assists to enhance the body's metabolic versatility. It additionally assists the body to adjust better to burning fat as a fuel source over the long-run.

Another significant aspect of carbohydrate cycling is how it permits insulin to be controlled. If you target your carbohydrates around your exercise, it can enhance your body's sensitivity to insulin. This signifies health. It assists in shielding versus conditions such as diabetes.

It additionally assists to optimize the many advantages that carbohydrates offer.

Is Carbohydrate Cycling Like Keto?

Many individuals believe that the keto eating plan and carbohydrate cycling are identical things. This isn't correct. Although there are some resemblances, the two programs are extremely different. The keto diet is very low in carbs. It additionally includes consuming a great deal of excellent fats and moderate quantities of protein. The primary objective of the keto diet plan is to burn fats as fuel by entering into ketosis.

Generally, carbohydrate cycling entails consuming more carbohydrates than you would have in the keto diet plan. It additionally does not entail consuming the identical quantity of fats. For that reason, ketosis isn't the goal of a carbohydrate cycling program.

However, there are some resemblances. Both highlight the management of carb consumption. Additionally, both eating plans include counting macros. Macros are the particular amounts of grams of proteins, fats and carbohydrates you consume every day. This suggests that some individuals integrate both programs. This is referred to as keto cycling.

The keto cycling procedure entails eating a keto diet plan on many days. These are going to be sprinkled with either a couple of days of eating more carbohydrates. These are referred to as refeeding days. They are developed to break the ketosis. By doing this, dieters can get the advantages of taking in carbs. Their fiber consumption is boosted, their athletic functionality is sustained, and their diet plan is more varied.

Some dietary professionals state that limiting carbohydrates in the long-term might impact specific hormones. Thyroid and insulin hormones are essential for healthy body structure.

If you attempt keto-cycling, the balance between these hormones might be much better kept. This supplies a unique benefit over the basic keto eating plan in which carbohydrates are limited over a prolonged duration. Not just that, however, the typical issues related to keto diet plans are removed or minimized. Problems like halitosis do not end up being widespread, given that some carbohydrates are still being taken in frequently.

Chapter 3: A Carbohydrate Cycling Diet Plan?

Carbohydrate cycling entails tracking macros with an app or a food journal. You need to figure out the amount of grams of carbs you'll have to consume daily. This might not be as simple as you thought. The quantity of carbohydrates you ought to consume is going to be particular to you. You have to bear numerous factors in mind. We'll look more carefully at those eventually. In the meantime, let's take a better look at what a typical carbohydrate cycling eating plan appears like.

High Carbohydrate Day

On a high carbohydrate day, you are going to typically acquire approximately 60 percent of your calories from complex carbs. That implies, if you're consuming approximately 1,500 calories daily, approximately 900 calories are complex carbohydrates.

If you're performing high-energy exercises such as interval training, sprints or long-distance running, you can include more carbohydrates. These ought to take the appropriate form though. You should not be including cake or donuts into your routine! Rather, you ought to offer yourself an extra serving of fruits, vegetables or whole grains.

The latter are all complex carbohydrates. This indicates they break down more gradually for a less quick release of energy. Simple carbohydrates such as sweets and cookies break down rapidly. This suggests that you obtain a super-fast energy rush followed by a crash. You ought to mostly consume complex carbs on a carbohydrate cycling routine. If you discover that you're having a hard time to handle your athletic exercises, attempt including another serving into your eating plan. You ought to just do this on days when you're going to the gym, though.

Low Carbohydrate Day

On days when you're not exercising or doing a relaxed workout, have a low carbohydrate day. On this type of day, you ought to substitute a number of your normal carbohydrate portions with veggies. You might additionally substitute a few of those carbohydrates with healthy proteins or fats.

Additionally, you might utilize a low-carb day as a beginning point from which to determine your high carbohydrate days. Typically, 50 grams of carbohydrates day-to-day suffices to reach ketosis. For that reason, you might start by taking in 50 grams of carbohydrates on low carbohydrate days. You can then advance from there, maxing out at 200 grams of carbohydrates daily.

Staying clear of the transactional food attitude is really crucial, nevertheless. Ideas such as "thirty minutes more running indicates that I can eat more carbohydrates" could be harmful. It causes an embroiled and challenging relationship with food and eating. However, consuming more carbohydrates some days with less carbohydrates on other days is how the body manages itself naturally. For that reason, decreasing carbohydrates offers advantages that you can make the most of.

A Week-Long Carbohydrate Cycling Program

The idea of carbohydrate cycling includes consuming very little carbohydrates for 2 days consecutively. This is going to be followed by a day of consuming more carbohydrates. There is a reason for this. When the reserves of carbohydrates are about to dry up, energy is restored thanks to a high carbohydrate day. This speeds up the metabolic process and causes more weight loss.

If you minimize your carbohydrates over 2 days, your fat stores are going to be utilized for energy. Your body is going to additionally go into a catabolic state. This suggests that the body begins to utilize muscle tissue to obtain energy from the proteins in your muscles.

It is necessary to understand what to consume over a week if you're preparing to carb cycle. Here is a sample seven-day strategy to guarantee you acquire all the important nutrients. You'll additionally get ample variety, so you do not get tired of your meals. If you can abide by this plan for 1 month, you ought to experience weight-loss advantages.

Day 1-- A Low Carbohydrate Day

Breakfast: Citrus and almond fruit salad blended with yogurt and berries.

Snack: Protein bar and an apple.

Lunch: Salad created with 100 grams of peas, 60 grams of quinoa, 2 hard-boiled eggs and tomatoes.

Snack: A scoop of walnuts and a banana.

Dinner: A sliced up stir-fried chicken breast with courgettes, chopped carrots, and green beans. Offered with 60 grams of quinoa.

Snack: 2 oatcakes.

Total Calories-- 1870

Total Carbs-- 224 grams

Total Proteins-- 106 grams

Total Fats-- 65 grams

Day 2-- Low Carbohydrate Day

Breakfast: Apple and seed muesli created with 2 tablespoons of rolled oats, sesame seeds, sunflower seeds, and pumpkin seeds. Offered with a little apple and 2 tablespoons of natural yogurt.

Snack: Scoop of walnuts and a banana.

Lunch: A whole meal pitta with a single tablespoon of cottage cheese, half an avocado, and tuna.

Snack: A pear.

Dinner: A grilled salmon steak with half a chopped lime on top. Offered with 60 grams of quinoa, 100 grams broccoli, and 70 grams of peas.

Snack: An apple.

Total Calories-- 1889

Total Carbs-- 160 grams

Total Proteins-- 130 grams

Total Fats-- 79 grams

Day 3-- High Carbohydrate Day

Breakfast: 50 grams of oats, submerged in water with 200 grams of berries. Offer with a tablespoon of sunflower seeds and a pot of organic yogurt.

Snack: A peach.

Lunch: A baked potato with a tablespoon of hummus. Offer with salad created from tomato, chopped cucumber, mixed leaves and red pepper.

Snack: An apple and a protein bar

Dinner: A grilled cod fillet offered with 100 grams of carrots, 250 grams of boiled potatoes, and peas.

Snack: 3 oatcakes.

Total Calories-- 1800

Total Carbs-- 320 grams

Total Proteins-- 80 grams

Total Fats—40 grams

Day 4-- Low Carbohydrate Day

Breakfast: 3 eggs beaten with 2 tablespoons of organic yogurt. Include half a courgette, half a red pepper, one tablespoon of peas and half an onion. Roast in a pan.

Snack: A small number of pumpkin seeds and an apple.

Lunch: A can of salmon combined with a can of butter beans. Offer with a salad of tomato, lettuce leaves, onion, and sugar snap peas.

Snack: A nectarine.

Dinner: A grilled turkey breast with carrot, grilled courgette, onion and red pepper.

Snack: 70 grams of grapes and a banana.

Total Calories—1810

Total Carbs-- 160 grams

Total protein-- 140 grams

Total fats-- 73 grams

Day 5-- Low Carbohydrate Day

Breakfast: 2 boiled eggs with 2 whole meal pitta pieces spread out with butter and marmite.

Snack: A pear and an apple.

Lunch: Tuna and avocado mash offered with salad leaves, tomato, cucumber, courgette and carrot.

Snack: A peace and an oatcake topped with cottage cheese and cucumber.

Dinner: A can of salmon combined with a can of sliced tomatoes, carrot, red pepper, tomato puree, and courgettes. Simmered for 10 minutes and offered.

Snack: A banana.

Total Calories—1800

Total Carbs-- 167 grams

Total Proteins-- 125 grams

Total Fats-- 78 grams

Day 6-- High Carbohydrate Day

Breakfast: 4 tablespoons of natural yogurt. Combine with 200 grams of berries, 50 grams of rolled oats, chopped pear and 1 tablespoon of honey.

Snack: An entire meal pitta bread packed with cottage cheese and a tomato.

Lunch: A chickpea salad with half a can of chickpeas.

Snack: 4 oatcakes with peanut butter and chopped apple.

Dinner: A grilled chicken breast with 60g quinoa, steamed broccoli, and 100g green beans.

Snack: A banana.

Total Calories-- 1850

Total Carbs-- 250 grams

Total Proteins-- 125 grams

Total Fats-- 45 grams

Day 7-- Low Carbohydrate Day

Breakfast: 2 poached eggs with 2 tomatoes and 2 portobello mushrooms.

Snack: A pot of organic yogurt, a peach and an orange.

Lunch: A pitta packed with avocado, cottage cheese, tomato, cucumber, peanut butter and lettuce.

Snack: An apple with a handful of pumpkin seeds and sunflower seeds.

Supper: Poached salmon with 200 grams tomatoes, a courgette, and sugar snap peas.

Snack: 2 oatcakes and a banana.

Total Calories-- 1825

Total Carbs-- 160 grams

Total Proteins-- 97 grams

Total Fats-- 95 grams

Chapter 4: Carbohydrate Cycling and Losing Weight

Carbohydrate cycling can assist with weight reduction by optimizing how the body utilizes fuel. When you embrace this eating plan, you consume less carbohydrates for 2 days, and then have a day of consuming more carbohydrates. How you alternate in between low and high carbohydrate days differs depending upon just how much activity you're doing. You take advantage of the carbohydrate fuel you obtain on the days when you're exercising. On the other hand, you gain from low carbohydrates if you're not active.

As you exercise, the body dips into its carb stores to discover energy. This implies you ought to line up high carbohydrate days with training days. This suggests your body can utilize the fuel to its finest advantage. It additionally implies that the extra energy permits you to exercise for longer. You'll, for that reason, burn more calories consequently. On days of rest, carbohydrates could be downsized. This is going to minimize the variety of empty calories you take in and assist you to slim down.

Imagine your weight is 170 pounds. You might intend to have 2 grams of carbohydrates for each pound of your weight on a high carbohydrate day. That would be approximately 340 grams. On low carbohydrate days, you might minimize this to approximately one gram per pound of your weight. This would take your carbohydrate consumption to 175 grams.

That does not indicate there's a set quantity of carbohydrates you can consume on each kind of day. Mainly, it depends upon what exercise you're doing. It additionally depends upon how often you're exercising. You'll discover a lot of suggestions online. Nevertheless, you'll have to customize your carb consumption to your own requirements.

Your metabolic process is going to increase or decrease depending upon your calorie and macronutrient consumption. If you consume sufficient carbohydrates at the appropriate time, your metabolic process is reset. This activates your body to discharge thyroid and leptin. These are hormones which control your body weight.

The standard American diet is extremely heavy in carbohydrates. This can generate an unfavorable impact, promoting the production of insulin frequently. Consequently, weight gain can happen, and conditions such as diabetes can establish. Low carbohydrate days urge your body to utilize all its glycogen (stashed carbohydrates). It shifts to burning ketones (body fat) as fuel. When kept fat is burned, weight is naturally shed.

Every carbohydrate cycling diet program is different. You have to select the one that meets your own objectives. A basic strategy is going to keep your carbohydrate consumption extremely low for 2 to 3 days. It is going to then boost your carbohydrate consumption for a day. That day ought to entail some rigorous activity.

On a low carbohydrate take, your carb consumption ought to be approximately between 50 grams and 150 grams. It ought to originate from non-starchy and dairy veggies. On a high carbohydrate day, you can have approximately 400 grams of carbohydrates. These can originate from starchy carbohydrates, and whole grains, in addition to non-starchy veggies and dairy.

Chapter 5: Additional Advantages of Carbohydrate Cycling

Carbohydrate cycling's main advantage is fast weight-loss. Nevertheless, there are some other advantages provided by doing this program that other diet plans do not offer. When you cycle in between low and high carbohydrate days, you reap the benefits provided by both kinds of dieting. Even better, a lot of the negatives of those diet plans are done away with.

A few of the advantages of carbohydrate cycling consist of enhanced insulin sensitivity. This assists to lower the threat of establishing type 2 diabetes. It can likewise enhance cholesterol levels and improve metabolic health. Anybody who is insulin resistant, pre-diabetic, or who has type 2 diabetes can gain from in this program.

Likewise, people who are resistant to weight loss might gain from this routine. By reducing carbohydrate consumption, insulin release is likewise lowered. This enables the body to burn quickly through carb stocks, changing to burning fat for energy. As a result, faster weight reduction could be set off.

Throughout the greater carbohydrate refeeding duration, hormones can delight in favorable results. Thyroid hormones, testosterone and leptin can all enjoy a positive effect. All these aspects have a crucial part to play in dieting success over the long-run. Hormones play an important part in workout effectiveness, metabolic process and craving management. For that reason, managing them more effectively is going to guarantee a much better function.

Chapter 6: Things to Remember

Carbohydrate cycling isn't an effort-free program. Lots of people start this routine without understanding just how much work is included. Preparation is crucial to your success. You have to count grams and weigh stuff in order to prosper. There are apps out there that can make life simpler. Nevertheless, if you desire a routine that is all planned out for you, carbohydrate cycling isn't for you. However, if standards and guidelines are your favored option, carbohydrate cycling is fantastic.

Are you considering giving it a try? Then keep reading to discover what you need to keep in mind when you do carb cycling.

Customize It To Your Liking

Your initial step is to make certain you get your carbohydrate cycling program right for you as a person. Everybody has various carbohydrate consumption requirements. That suggests there's no single one-size-fits-all option. You'll have to figure out your own everyday calorie target for each day. This could be difficult.

One typical method is:

- Wish to slim down? Multiply your weight by 10. This is the amount of calories you ought to take in every day.

- Wish to preserve your current weight? Multiply your weight by 12. This is the amount of calories you'll have to consume daily.

- Wish to put on weight? Multiply your weight by 15. This is the number of calories you'll have to consume daily.

When you know the amount of calories to go for, it's time to carry on to the following step.

You have to split up those calories among the 3 primary macronutrients: protein, fats and carbs. Carbohydrates and proteins both supply 4 calories for each gram. Fats offer 9 calories per gram. In addition to carbohydrate cycling, you ought to go for approximately one gram of protein for every pound of your weight. The remainder ought to be comprised of healthy fats.

On a high carbohydrate day, you'll increase the amount of carbohydrates you consume. You'll likewise boost your calorie consumption. The protein and fat levels are going to stay the identical. On low carbohydrate days, you'll decrease your calorie consumption. Once again, your protein and fat levels are going to stay the identical. Basically, carbohydrate cycling has to do with lowering your calorie consumption, while not feeling as if you are lowering it.

It is essential to bear in mind that if you keep your carbohydrates too low for a number of days, you can experience ill-effects. Carbohydrate cravings, sleep issues, tiredness, irritation, bloating, irregularity and bad mood can all happen consequently. This takes place due to the fact that your body has actually consumed all its carbs and is changing to utilizing fat as fuel. It's a phenomenon referred to as "carbohydrate flu." It is momentary, however, if you preserve your hydration level and take in ample electrolytes, it'll pass rapidly.

Not everybody can deal with carbohydrate cycling programs, however. For some individuals, it's a counter-productive method to eat. Individuals struggling with Hashimoto's or who have adrenal fatigue can discover their thyroid hormone creation is decreased. This can decrease their metabolic rate and induce weight gain. Individuals who are breastfeeding, pregnant, have a background of eating disorders or who are currently underweight ought to stay clear of this program.

Protein and Calories

When you're carb cycling, it could be appealing to remove a great deal of things from your eating plan. It is necessary to bear in mind that it's just refined carbohydrates that have to be slashed.

When you're consuming less carbohydrates, you have to make sure that fiber is a crucial part of your diet plan. A low carbohydrate day isn't a reason to neglect broccoli or apples. Mostly, concentrate on getting sugar and simple carbohydrates from your eating plan. Muffins and bagels can go. Nutrient-rich, fiber-filled foods such as quinoa, beans, oats, veggies and fruits ought to all remain.

If you focus on high-fiber carbs on your low carbohydrate days, you'll feel more satiated. Your cholesterol levels are going to be much better managed, and your microbiome is going to be healthier. This is going to assist you to handle your weight successfully given that you will not be lured to binge. Swelling is going to additionally be minimized, assisting to fight weight problems.

You might believe you can shed more weight if you decrease your calorie consumption considerably. Nevertheless, you still have to eat sufficiently. Even on a low carbohydrate day, you have to keep proper calorie consumption.

The brain needs carbs to operate. Particularly, it needs glucose to run efficiently. If there is no glucose for it to utilize, the body needs to utilize another source. It might wind up utilizing protein for this function. This is horrible news when you wish to build up and preserve lean muscle. You need, for that reason, to eat over 120 grams of carbohydrates even on a low carbohydrate day. The brain requires to be fed, so you do not spend the entire day walking in a fog.

Bear in mind that the quality of the food you consume matters just as much as the quantity. Your high carb days should not be loaded with pizza and french fries! You ought to delight in whole grains rather. Bread, whole grain pasta and brown rice are much healthier choices than refined sugars.

If you aren't certain what you ought to be consuming, you ought to speak with a specialist. The quantity of carbohydrates that you'll require is going to differ depending upon your composition. It is going to differ depending upon your calorific requirements, your activity level and the kind of workout you do. It'll additionally differ depending upon your weight, height and gender. A diet professional can assist to offer you a tailored suggestion. This is going to guarantee you have the ability to get the correct amount of fuel you need to optimize your outcomes.

Chapter 7: Carbohydrate Cycling Types

Carbohydrate cycling exemplifies a technique to dieting in which carbohydrate consumption is rotated. There are no set guidelines about the basis on which you perform this. Some individuals alternate every day, while others alternate on a month-to-month or weekly basis. Some individuals do extended periods of high, moderate and low carbohydrate diet plans. Others change their technique on a day to day basis.

This indicates that there is no single kind of carbohydrate cycling to fit everybody. Everybody ought to configure their carbohydrate consumption. They may do this to match a variety of aspects. These consist of:

- Your own body structure objectives

- Your arranged refeeds

- Your training and rest days

- Whether you're participating in a competition.

- The kind of training you're performing and its magnitude

- Your body fat level

Some carbohydrate cycling approaches entail 2 days of low carbohydrates followed by a day of high carbohydrates. This pattern repeats.

Another technique is to have 2 days of high carbohydrate consumption, followed by 2 days of mild carbohydrates. There are going to then be 3 days of low carbohydrates prior to going back to the start of the cycle. Typically, the protein consumption is going to stay comparable in between all days. Fat consumption, on the other hand, is going to differ depending upon the consumption of carbs. High carb days generally indicate low-fat. Low carbohydrate days indicate high fat.

Another method entails changing your carbohydrate consumption week on week. For instance, you might consume a low carbohydrate diet plan for 11 days in a row. You might then have high carbohydrates for the following 3 days prior to going back to the start of the cycle.

There is even a regular monthly change method. This includes consuming low carbohydrates for 4 weeks, and after that, having a week of high carbohydrates for the 5th week. As you can see, there are numerous variations of carbohydrate cycling. That indicates that some trial and error and individual experimentation are going to be needed. In time, you'll ultimately discover the best formula to fit you.

A short summary of a few of the most typical carbohydrate cycling methods is as follows:

- An irregular, big refeed. This includes increasing carbohydrate consumption once in one to two weeks throughout a low carbohydrate consumption stage.

- Moderate regular refeeds. This entails increasing carbohydrate consumption every 3 to 4 days in a low carbohydrate consumption stage.

- Strategic carbohydrate cycling. This includes structuring menus with a moderate carbohydrate consumption at particular, strategic periods in a low carbohydrate consumption stage. When you follow this technique, you'll steer far from extremely high carbohydrate consumption. It is going to, for that reason, permit your metabolic process to catch up to your dietary consumption.

- Carbohydrate cycling to build muscle. Anybody who wishes to gain muscle mass is going to need a calorie surplus. Nevertheless, when you over-consume calories in the long-run, body fat gain is practically unavoidable. Carbohydrate cycling permits muscle gain to be enhanced over fat gain. Like strategic carbohydrate cycling, menus need to be prepared to suit your weekly schedule. This is going to allow you to make a short-term excess of calories to improve lean mass and strength gains.

Chapter 8: Which Foods Are Should You Be Eating?

Prior to starting a carbohydrate cycling routine, you have to understand more about what carbohydrates are. You likewise have to understand which ones appropriate to consume on this kind of diet plan. Carbs typically have unfavorable associations. Nevertheless, not all carbohydrates are bad for you. Carbs are vital in providing energy. Here, we take a closer look at which ones you ought to be taking pleasure in as part of your carbohydrate cycling way of life.

Carbs That Are Good For You

Along with proteins and fats, carbohydrates are among the 3 primary macronutrients. Carbohydrates are required to provide energy to the body and brain. Whenever you consume carbohydrates, they're broken down throughout food digestion into sugars. These sugars are then taken in into the blood stream. In reaction to the increase in blood glucose levels, the body launches insulin. It is required to transport the sugar (referred to as glucose at this phase) to the cells. This permits a fast energy increase to fuel activity. Carbohydrates likewise get saved in the muscles and liver as glycogen. This is a saved kind of glucose. Nevertheless, excess glucose likewise gets saved as fat. For that reason, a great deal of individuals believe that carbs are harmful.

Not all carbs are equivalent. There are 3 main kinds of carbs: fiber, sugar and starch. Sugar is, without a doubt, the least complex type. Starch and fiber are both complex carbs. This suggests they are harder to break down in the body. It takes longer, and for that reason, you'll feel satiated for longer when you consume complex carbohydrates. Refined or processed carbs are less starchy and fibrous. They are sweeter and have less dietary worth.

Processed carbohydrates could be dumped from your diet plan when you're carb cycling. Nevertheless, whole foods that are abundant in carbohydrates ought to remain in your diet plan. Potatoes and starchy veggies like squash and carrots are complex carbs which are great for you. Whole grains like quinoa and brown rice and legumes like beans and lentils are additionally excellent options. Even foods consisting of natural sugars like fruit and milk have a place in carbohydrate cycling diet plans.

These wholefoods have dietary benefits. They include crucial vitamins and minerals. For that reason, although the word carbs typically generates images of sweet food that is unhealthy, this isn't constantly the case. Complex carbohydrates have an important function to play in guaranteeing you have a healthy way of life.

Naturally, that does not imply that all carbs could be featured in a carbohydrate cycling eating plan. Some ought to constantly be avoided other than as periodic snacks. Yet there are great deals of healthy sources of carb which have great deals of helpful minerals, fiber and vitamins. They additionally taste terrific. For that reason, when planning a high carbohydrate menu, you should not see it as a reason to binge on cookies. Rather, place your concentration on healthy complex carbohydrate options.

Some good carbs consist are:

- Wholegrains-- unmodified grains have lots of health advantages. They're extremely healthy and consist of oats, quinoa and brown rice.

- Veggies-- all veggies have various vitamin and mineral material. You ought to consume several colors to get the best balance.

- Unprocessed fruit-like veggies, all fruits are distinct. Berries are particularly healthy, considering that they have a high antioxidant material and a low glycemic index.

- Legumes-- these complex carbohydrates are absorbed gradually. They are loaded with fiber and minerals.

- Tubers-- white and sweet potatoes are additionally complex carbohydrates. They are gradually absorbed so you'll feel satiated for longer.

How do you recognize which carbs are good ones? They are going to be:

- High in fiber

- Slow to absorb

- Unprocessed without any natural components taken out

Bad carbohydrates, on the other hand, are going to be:

- Discovered in really processed foods
- Including white flour
- High in sugar
- Low in fiber

What would be great examples of carbohydrates to eat at each phase of your carbohydrate cycling program?

On a no-carb day you ought to consume:

- Veggies that are high in fiber such as leafy greens, mushrooms, asparagus, and broccoli
- Good fats
- Lean protein

You ought to stay clear of consuming:

- Starchy carbohydrates. These consist of oats, potatoes, rice and cereal. They additionally consist of starchy veggies such as squash, zucchini, pumpkin, and beans. Your overall consumption of carbohydrates ought to be beneath 25 grams each day. All of these ought to originate from fiber-filled veggies.

On low carbohydrate days, you ought to consume:

- Fibrous veggies

- 2 to 3 portions of starch. All ought to be from sources such as brown rice, sweet potatoes, fruit, oats and starchy veggies. They ought to be devoid of soy, dairy and gluten. Starchy carbohydrates ought to be consumed after your exercise for the very best outcomes.

On high carb days, you ought to consume:

- Approximately 200 grams of carbohydrates for a woman or 300 grams for a male. The overall quantity is going to differ to fit your size and activity level.

- A lot of healthy fats.

- A great deal of lean protein.

High carb days should not be a reason for binge eating. They are a means of methodically resetting your muscle-building and fat-burning hormones. The majority of the fats ought to be from a clean source. Nevertheless, if you're about to cheat, ensure to do it on one of these high carbohydrate days.

There are mistaken beliefs that foods such as pasta are banned from carbohydrate cycling eating plans. This isn't always correct. If you place any food off-limits, you'll simply wish to binge on it more. You can have foods such as pasta.

Nevertheless, if you intend to consume starchy foods that have little micronutrients and fiber, you'll have to consume them carefully. You ought to just have them after you have actually exercised. This is since your insulin sensitivity is going to be greatest at that time. Your body is going to, for that reason, have the ability to utilize them at their finest at this time. They're less probable to be transformed into fat in the body and stocked.

On a high carbohydrate day, your focus ought to stay on complex carbohydrates. You ought to stay clear of simple carbohydrates. Complex carbs assist you to remain satiated for longer. They all consist of more vitamins and nutrients. On a no-carb day, you can't simply eliminate sugar and starch, however. You have to substitute those absent calories which you 'd normally derive from carbohydrates with something else. Good fats are an excellent replacement.

Obviously, not all fats are great fats. Carbohydrate cycling is distinct from a keto diet plan. In the keto way of life, consuming all fats is urged. Even sources of saturated fat like bacon and cheese can be consumed openly. On a carbohydrate cycling routine, these sources ought to be kept away from. Good fats that are concentrated on omega-3 fats could be consumed openly. You can discover these in healthy sources like chia seeds, avocados, fish and olives.

Specialists frequently suggest medium-chain triglycerides like MCT oil on a carbohydrate cycling routine. These promote your neurological functions even on days when you're not consuming carbohydrates. Along with good fats, you ought to ensure to consume a lot of lean proteins. Proteins consist of no carbs. For that reason, it could be consumed openly even on a no-carb day. Lean chicken, eggs and fish are all excellent options. They are going to assist you to feel satiated while increasing muscle development.

Chapter 9: Sample Programs

As we have actually currently explained, there are lots of types of carbohydrate cycling program. This makes it difficult to choose how you're going to set about starting. If you're prepared to put a carbohydrate cycling program of your own in place, here are some sample programs. They are going to assist you to choose what works ideally for you.

2 of the most prominent programs are The High/Low Programand The High/Medium/Low Program.

Let's take a look at the High/Low Program initially. This approach entails having a high carb day, and then a low carbohydrate day. A high carb day entails consuming more than 150 grams of carbohydrates. A low carb day entails consuming less than 100 grams of carbohydrates. The specific requirements and measurements are going to differ to fit each dieter. Nevertheless, let's picture we're preparing a program for a 28-year-old male. Envision he weighs 185 pounds and is 5 feet 8 inches high. The overall amount of calories he requires to preserve weight is 185 x 15 i.e. 2775. He additionally weight trains 3 days a week. We're going to take a look at a couple of programs to fit his data to meet various targets.

First of all, let's take a look at an appropriate program for him if he wished to lose fat. With this objective in mind, he would require 3 days of high carbs. These would be at the level of calories needed for upkeep. He would then follow this up with 4 days of low carbohydrate eating. These 4 days would all be 600 calories beneath this upkeep figure. He would select his 3 weightlifting days as his high carb days. His non-workout days would be his low carb days.

His program would, for that reason, look something like this:

Training day consumption-- 2775 calories

Protein consumption-- 185 g

Carbohydrate consumption-- 370 g

Fat consumption-- 70 g

Day of rest consumption-- 2175 calories

Protein consumption-- 185 g

Carbohydrate consumption-- 100 g

Fat consumption-- 110 g

His overall deficit of calories each week would be 600 x 4 i.e. 2400 calories. This would assist him to lose almost 1 pound of fat each week. While this might not sound remarkable, it is essential to bear in mind that quick weight loss isn't the only objective. The faster the fat is lost, the higher the likelihood of losing muscle too. This is the reverse of the purpose of carbohydrate cycling.

What if the identical person wished to attempt carbohydrate cycling to build up muscle? In this case, his calorie consumption has to be changed somewhat. He requires a surplus of calories in this circumstance. This is going to assist him to recuperate after exercising. It'll likewise promote more muscle tissue development. His objective is to have a surplus of 300 calories on his training days. On his low carbohydrate days, he'll remain at his advised upkeep consumption. His program would, for that reason, appear like this:

Training day consumption-- 3075 calories

Protein consumption-- 185 g

Carbohydrate consumption-- 430 g

Fat consumption-- 80 g

Day of rest consumption-- 2775 calories

Protein consumption-- 185 g

Carbohydrate consumption-- 300 g

Fat consumption-- 90 g

You'll most likely see that the carbohydrate consumption on a low carbohydrate day is remarkably high. Previously, we stated the carbohydrate consumption on a low carbohydrate day ought to be beneath 100 grams. Yet, in this case, the person has a high energy output. For that reason, staying clear of excess fat is essential. Fat could be kept quickly when there's a calorie surplus. For that reason, staying clear of consuming excessive fat is necessary to protect against fat gain. On the other hand, carbohydrates are necessary to fill up muscle glycogen and promote recuperation. This helps in training efficiency.

With this program, the person is cycling carbohydrates, yet, not so considerably as he would in order to reduce weight. Some individuals discover that keeping carbohydrate consumption under 100g on their low carbohydrate days assists them to remain leaner. Nevertheless, calorie consumption needs to be kept at an identical level in general, even on off days. This is going to make sure a net calorie surplus is kept over the whole week.

The high/medium/low approach? Well, this entails having a high carb day, and then a medium carbohydrate day. Lastly, a low carb day is going to follow. The cycle is going to then restart. A high carb day includes consuming more than 150 grams of carbohydrates. A medium carbohydrate day includes consuming in between 100 grams and 150 grams of carbohydrates. A low carb day includes consuming less than 50 grams of carbohydrates.

Now, let's picture our dieter. She's a 30-year-old woman who is 5 feet 5 inches tall. She weighs 155 pounds and exercises 3 days each week doing weightlifting. Her overall calories for upkeep are 155 x 15 (2325).

If she wishes to shed fat, this is a sample carbohydrate cycling program for her.She ought to have 2 days of high carbohydrate consumption. The calorie consumption is going to be set at her upkeep level of 2325 calories. On her 2 medium carbohydrate days, her calorie consumption is going to be 300 calories under this level. On her 2 low carbohydrate days, her calorie consumption is going to be 600 calories beneath her upkeep level. Instead of lining up the high carb days with her training days, the consumption is: staggered. Training ought to be performed on high and medium carbohydrate days, however, not on low carbohydrate days.

Her program is going to, for that reason, appear like this:

High carbohydrate day consumption-- 2325 calories

Protein consumption-- 150 g

Carbohydrate consumption-- 250 g

Fat consumption-- 80 g

Medium carbohydrate day consumption-- 2025 calories

Protein consumption-- 150 g

Carbohydrate consumption-- 140 g

Fat consumption-- 80 g

Low carbohydrate day consumption-- 1725 calories

Protein consumption-- 150 g

Carbohydrate consumption-- 60 g

Fat consumption-- 100 g

Over the week, the strategy might appear like this:

Monday-- high carbohydrate-- training day

Tuesday-- medium carbohydrate-- training day

Wednesday--low carbohydrate-- day of rest

Thursday-- high carbohydrate-- training day

Friday-- medium carbohydrate-- day of rest

Saturday-- low carbohydrate-- day of rest

Sunday-- low carbohydrate-- day of rest

If the identical person wished to gain muscle through carbohydrate cycling, the program would appear different. A calorie surplus is going to be needed so that muscle tissue can recuperate and grow. For that reason, a 200-calorie surplus is going to be needed on a training day. On day of rest, she ought to consume the amount of calories needed for upkeep.

Her program is going to, for that reason, be like this:

High carbohydrate day consumption-- 2525 calories

Protein consumption-- 150 g

Carbohydrate consumption-- 350 g

Fat consumption-- 60 g

Medium carbohydrate day consumption-- 2525 calories

Protein consumption-- 150 g

Carbohydrate consumption-- 250 g

Fat consumption-- 90 g

Low carbohydrate day consumption-- 2325 calories

Protein consumption-- 150 g

Carbohydrate consumption-- 140 g

Fat consumption-- 120 g

You might have seen the medium carbohydrate day requirement is greater than recommended previously. The identical factors apply in this case as used in the above instance. Consuming too much dietary fat in such situations can result in the storage of fat. For that reason, staying clear of consuming excessive fat assists to prevent fat gain. Carbohydrates are crucial in healing and in filling up the muscle glycogen. This assists to improve training functionality.

The person in question here is still carb cycling. Nevertheless, her strategy isn't as extreme as it would be if she wished to lose fat. If you utilize this technique to build muscle mass, you can change the fat and carbohydrate numbers to match you.

Some individuals discover that if they keep their carbs to under 100g on a day of rest, they remain leaner. This might work for you, however, you'll still require for your calorie consumption to stay at the upkeep level even on a day of rest. This is going to guarantee that you remain in a calorie surplus overall throughout the week.

The crucial nutrient for gaining and preserving muscle is protein. Nonetheless, it does not need to be incredibly high, whether you wish to build muscle or decrease fat, 1g of protein for every pound of your bodyweight is perfect. Carbohydrate and fat totals are essential too. Nevertheless, they could be customized to your energy expense and choices.

How about if you wish to preserve your bodyweight? You can still accomplish this objective with carbohydrate cycling. You merely have to select one of the above approaches. You then calibrate training day and rest day consumptions, so they balance out over the week. One method of accomplishing this is to take in 200 calories more than your suggested upkeep level on a training day. On a day of rest, you ought to have 200 calories under this figure. So, if your upkeep consumption is 2400 calories, you'd have 2600 on training days and 2300 on a day of rest.

Chapter 10: How to Begin

Although the concept of carbohydrate cycling is enticing, it's hard to know how to begin. This program could be rather complicated. For that reason, you have to know as much as feasible about carbs and how they operate in the body. You likewise have to comprehend how to pick the appropriate carbohydrate cycling program for you. The info we have actually supplied in the earlier chapters is going to assist you to figure out the best program for you. Nevertheless, you might most likely gain from a couple of professional ideas to get you off to the best start. Here is some excellent guidance to point you in the appropriate direction.

Initially, we'll take a look at how to stay clear of the significant mistakes of carbohydrate cycling. Here are a few of the most typical ones:

- Focusing exclusively on carbohydrates while disregarding other macros. Some individuals are puzzled by the name "carbohydrate cycling." It's a misnomer. Carbohydrate cycling isn't just about carbs. It has to do with stabilizing your calorie consumption over the week. If carbohydrate consumptions are reduced on a day of rest, more fats and proteins have to be consumed to compensate. It's just by doing this that weight loss could be preserved in the long run.

You have to understand how many calories you have to take in to preserve weight initially. This allows you to plan just how much you have to change your consumption to match each training or rest day. On a day of rest, take between 10 and 20 percent off your calorie consumption from carbs, however, do not boost your fat or protein consumption. There are 4 calories in every gram of carb. For that reason, if you consume 2000 calories every day, cut your consumption of carbohydrates by 50 grams on day of rest.

- Your calorie consumption is differing excessively. The 10 to 20 percent guideline particularly applies to carbohydrates. Nevertheless, you should not ever have more than a 33 percent distinction in the overall quantity of calories taken in over the week. Excessive difference harms recuperation. It likewise makes it harder to follow the carbohydrate cycling routine. You can correct this by consuming a minimum of 68 percent of your normal energy consumption on low carbohydrate days.

- You're utilizing your high carbohydrate days as a cheat day. High output days aren't a reason to consume anything you want. If you do this frequently, unhealthy eating behaviors begin to set in. You can repair this by concentrating primarily on foods that are dense in nutrients.

Consume more whole foods like potatoes and oats on your high carbohydrate days. Consume more eggs and nuts on your low carbohydrate days. You'll feel satiated and you will not destroy your total regimen.

Now you understand what to stay clear of, here are some suggestions for each carbohydrate cycling program.

- Base your picked dietary approach on your basal calorie requirements and activity levels.

- Pick your refeed days well beforehand.

- Constantly follow your routine up until your refeeding day.

- Keep all your decisions based upon the result. Various techniques for refeeding work best for different body types. You ought to take body composition tests to make sure you're on the greatest track for you.

- Work out on your refeeding days. This is going to guarantee the ideal body composition outcomes.

- On refeed days, consume more carbohydrates in the early morning and during times when you're performing a great deal of physical activity.

- On low carb days, consume extra leafy greens. They are practically devoid of calories; however, include more bulk to your plate. You'll discover a full-looking plate to be more rewarding.

- Consume whole food fats on low carbohydrate days. Coldwater fish, grass-fed butter, eggs, nuts, coconut oil, and avocado are all great options.

- Measure your fats and carbohydrates. This is going to assist you to monitor the number of calories you take in. On a regular day, determine your carbohydrates too. A great deal of the time, we ignore just how much protein we're consuming and overstate the quantity of carbohydrates and fat.

- Do not lower carbohydrates without consuming more fat. Your body needs either carbohydrates or fats for energy. That suggests you'll have to fuel up for the day in one way or the other.

- Avoid skipping meals. You may be lured to stay away from eating to drop more weight on typical or low carbohydrate days. This is a horrible idea. It might lead to your body breaking down extra muscle.

- Stay clear of winging it. Choosing to attempt carbohydrate cycling is really different than actually doing it. You'll have to be committed and keep in-depth records of your consumption at each meal. You'll have to do this daily for weeks on end. There's no chance to take a look at an active ingredient and understand its macronutrient and calorie contents. For that reason, you'll have to measure appropriately. Apps like MyFitnessPal and MyPlate are great for this.

- Constantly pick foods that support your total wellness, even on high carbohydrate days. Substantial mounds of white bread and pasta, gallons of sweet beverages and lots of cake will not assist your health. Choose complex carbohydrates that are abundant in fiber. Wholegrain bread, quinoa and oatmeal are all pleasing and filling. They're likewise great for your health.

- Indulge sometimes. Even if you ought to be eating healthily the majority of the time, that does not indicate you can never ever indulge. If you prohibited yourself from consuming bagels or desserts, you'll simply wind up craving them. Because of this, you'll wind up cheating more and destroying your diet plan. It might likewise result in a harmful relationship with food and eating with time. If you select complex carbohydrates on many high carbohydrate days, you can have the occasional candy bar or cookie.

- Speak with a professional. Nutrition could be a complex topic, nuanced for everybody. Working carefully with an expert could, for that reason, be an excellent idea. A nutritional expert is going to have the ability to prepare an individualized diet program which is based upon your requirements. It is going to be customized to match your situation, your activity level and your goals. This is going to guarantee you get all the appropriate nutrients, while still attaining your selected results.

Conclusion

As you can see, there are numerous benefits related to carbohydrate cycling. Nonetheless, it isn't a diet plan program for everybody. You have to be dedicated to persevere.

Carbohydrate cycling is perfect for anybody who understands what they wish to attain from their diet plan. There are a couple of things you have to do prior to you getting going, however. You'll have to understand your upkeep calorie consumption. This is going to be based upon your activity level, age, gender, and height. When you have this figure, you have to match it with your preferred result. It's then reasonably easy to figure out the ideal plan for you.

Whether you wish to gain muscle, lose weight or both, carbohydrate cycling can be perfect for you. If you have actually just recently dropped weight and wish to preserve it, it's likewise helpful for you. You merely have to pick the ideal carbohydrate cycling program to fit your schedule. Align your low and high carbohydrate days with your activity level and physique objectives. You can then utilize the info supplied in this book to select appropriate foods for you.

Bear in mind that you have to select the ideal dietary consumption daily when you're carb cycling. You can't simply delight in starchy and sweet foods when you feel like it. While you can have a periodic snack, you generally have to concentrate on eating complex carbohydrates. Making certain to keep your fat and protein consumption level consistent each day of the week is likewise essential.

With the appropriate method, you might discover that carbohydrate cycling is the weight reduction answer you have been searching for all along.

I hope that you enjoyed reading through this book and that you have found it useful. If you want to share your thoughts on this book, you can do so by leaving a review on the Amazon page. Have a great rest of the day.

Printed in Great Britain
by Amazon